Table of Contents

The Efficacy of Face Masks in Filtering Allergens

The Efficacy of Face Masks in Managing Allergies

1. Introduction to Allergies and Face Masks

Allergic people could benefit from this information so that they can wear face masks if needed and take other precautions to limit their exposure to airborne triggers and manage their allergic symptoms. It is widely known that air filtration systems with high-efficiency particulate air (HEPA) filters can manage allergy symptoms, but the efficacy of using DIY masks or face masks bought without a prescription for the management of allergies is largely unknown. Some face masks are available on prescription. These face masks are backed by scientific evidence regarding efficiency in trapping airborne particles and their impact on a person's quality of life and/or their allergic symptomology.

Face masks are used in clinical settings to protect patients from the mucus that is released during surgical or clinical procedures and to protect healthcare workers from any infections that may be transmitted through the mucus. The masks are also worn by the general public to prevent infection from diseases such as COVID-19. Now, the general public is also wearing them to manage hay fever. Face masks are effective at trapping airborne particles that can cause symptoms of allergies in pollen and dust mite sensitized people.

Allergies are a common occurrence, with as many as one in three people showing symptoms at some point in their lives due to a genetic component. Some of the most common allergic sensitivities are to pollen, dust mites, or pets, which affect the eyes and nasal passages, causing flu-like symptoms such as sneezing and, in some cases, asthma. In the United Kingdom, 20% of people are allergic to pets, while 300 million people in the world are allergic to grass pollen.

2. Types of Face Masks

2. Surgical Masks: are designed to help protect the sterile field from particles, blood, splashes, sprays, or splatter that may contain germs (viruses and bacteria) that may spread infection. They have limited ability to protect bigger particles from getting through the material due to the loose fit and do not help protect against chemicals or gases in the air. Individuals who are allergic to various things might also use a surgical face mask during high-pollen times. Moreover, both disposable and reusable surgical masks can be worn. Cloth surgical face masks may be put on over the ears and attached in the back of the head with twine. Many adults prefer a surgical mask for comfort because it is less visible than a respirator. Filters do come within the mask, but individuals can cut a coffee filter or HEPA filter lining to shape. People receiving layer masks have the potential of catching germs on the water droplets included by the carrier.

1. N95 Respirators: are used to protect the wearer from airborne particles and from liquid contaminating the face. They filter out at least 95% of very small (0.3 micron) particles. They are used to control germ transfers, and they also protect against pollen, pet dander, dust mites, and other allergens. Only those individuals who work in a high-pollen area wear N95s. High-quality N95 masks can filter the vast majority of small particles ranging from 0.5 to 0.3 micrometres. They are relatively expensive and may be reused, but they must first be cleansed with soap and

water, bleach, or alcohol. Moreover, a half facepiece can cost as little as $15.00.

Face masks are typically used to filter the air that we breathe, helping to reduce the number of allergens that may penetrate the nose and mouth. According to a community-based study published in The Journal of Allergy and Clinical Immunology, the efficacy of different types of face masks in combating allergies has been rather low. However, there are currently three types of masks that may be worn as prophylactic or treatment intervention for various allergies.

2.1. N95 Respirators

The N95 respirator mask is made of a material that blocks 95% of solid and liquid aerosol, as well as certain non-oil-based particles. N95 masks have several physical layers that help protect you from allergies, including one layer of an absorbent layer of an aqueous layer, a moisture-wicking covering, and other non-woven fabric layers. No air valves are packaged. Masks can be worn for more than 8 hours. It can be highly effective when managing allergies. However, they can affect younger honey breeders over time who are not accustomed to using protective gear.

Masks: The most significant aspect is breathing protection, as it characterizes the type of mask that will greatly reduce the inhalation of dust, bacteria, and so on. N95 respirators can be approved in the US through various routes, such as NIOSH. They are subject to stringent testing to measure filtration efficiency, such as collection efficiency for NaCl and DOP, as well as 42 CFR 84 approval procedures. As these respirators have a particulate filter, they can be tested for fit for liquid or oily-based aerosol. It is also worth noting that the price of N95 respirators can be higher compared to regular medical masks, commonly known as facemasks, although people still prefer N95 quality as preferred. In case of allergies, asthma, and other related problems, you should use only N95 respirators to provide greater protection and to avoid costly asthma treatments.

2.2. Surgical Masks

During an active pollen season, the pollen that is floating in the air in Central Europe is measured in the millions per cubic meter. In a compact car moving 1km on an open highway with the air system turned off, the entire cabin will fill with air that measures several thousand pollen per cubic meter. Given the size of the pollen in comparison with the gaps in the design of a surgical mask, I believe there might be some benefit in the case of ocular allergies and hives, but I do tend to be skeptical of the overall benefit in reducing allergic rhinitis with the use of a surgical face mask.

Back To Basics: Surgical masks are not capable of closing around the mouth and nose, which, in turn, means that air will always flow around the filter. This can lead to a tighter fit in the ear loops and pressure on the face from the mask. If you have tried wearing one, even for a few minutes, you can appreciate how much heat you must generate in order for the mask to even feel a little damp on the inside.

Surgical masks are a medical product that was intended for the protection of sterile fields of use by preventing drops of body fluids from coming into contact with wounds and sterile bandages. When it comes to pollen and other allergens, a surgical mask will filter out the larger allergens and, in doing so, might help a sensitive person in reducing the total allergen exposure. This, in turn, might help in raising the person's trigger threshold.

2.3. Cloth Masks

However, these qualities can be considered separately or in combination due to the possibility of anaphylaxis. For definitions of allergens and particles, pieces, species, grains, or biological entities in aeroplankton (apportioned into aerobes and anaerobes) see Table 1 and enterobes (at least in transition to aeroplancton) see Table 2. For correspondence in general botanical terms, see Table 3.

To evaluate mask efficacy and guide individuals wisely, it is important to consider the following elements and how they apply to allergic responses: 1. Size of particle removed and its impact on the wearer; 2. The composition of the particle and the wearer's sensitivity to it; 3. The removal of particles and the conditions that enhance, reduce, or render non-functional such an approach, and; 4. The psychological and social impacts of wearing a face covering, as humans are among some of the most elaborate social signals in the animal kingdom.

2.3.1. Characteristics of Cloth Masks Cloth masks are made of multiple layers, where the primary function of cotton, silk, or another fiber is to avoid disrupting allergens during use. The major advantage of a cloth mask is that if the wearer feels an imminent exposure, such as a dust cloud, smoothing the mask from the outside could increase the mask's efficiency at that moment.

Our focus in this section is on cloth masks, which have different characteristics than surgical masks (more commonly referred to as 'face masks' throughout this paper). These images of cloth masks are for demonstration purposes only; the mask colors shown are not necessarily recommended.

3. Mechanism of Action

Face masks can help alleviate nasal allergy symptoms, and masks can be used whenever you are away from home. They can also be used when cutting the grass or doing housework that involves dust. Durable wood or metal, plastic, foam, or canister respirators are good options if allergy symptoms occur away from home. Use air purifiers and air cleaners in your home if indoor allergens such as mold, dust, or pet dander trigger nasal symptoms. Face masks are essential for health workers, teachers, or students during fire season to protect them from smoke in the environment. Face masks help reduce the inhalation of irritating and harmful allergens and make breathing easier. One option for a face mask is a paper mask, while another option is a cloth mask as it is more comfortable and reusable. Certain cloth masks have inserts for filters to maximize effectiveness. The key is in the flexibility and moisture-wicking ability of the fabric. Mask resistance, breathability, and a moldable nose bridge are all good features to have.

Face masks for allergies can help reduce the effects of allergy symptoms that are triggered when allergens are inhaled. These masks are designed to filter allergens from the air that you inhale. The allergens do not accumulate on the surface of the mask; the material used is designed to attract the allergen and keep it away from your respiratory tract. Although there are several breathing apparatuses that can help those who suffer from asthma and allergies, we will focus on face masks that are available in the market according to their respective specifications. The fibers can attract and retain allergens, and negative ions are used in the inner layer of the mask. Some face masks are simply paper or fleece masks with no special capabilities. Surgical masks are designed to be worn by health professionals to protect against potentially dangerous substances. Masks designed to avoid dust or for industrial use are also useful in reducing dust and pollen.

3.1. Filtration of Allergens

The aim of this section is to show that even in the absence of any clinical controls or actual clinical evidence, under laboratory conditions, we found that face masks reduced the amounts of allergen particles trapped in testing chambers. However, allergies are not entirely comprised of microorganisms. Also, allergies are widely considered as critical problems, perhaps making this filter function of face masks their most critical aspect. Please note that in case studies, when allergies are secondary to infectious complications such as fungal sinusitis, many more microorganisms attached to allergen-denuded filters are retrieved. Thus, the microorganisms in the collection are consistent with the focus of the filter aspect.

Filtration is a critical item that masks are employed for, using various forms of fabrics, including non-electrostatic breadcloths and electrostatic charging polypropylene. It is well known that the reason face masks are believed to be potentially useful in reducing the exposure to pollen and spores is due to the filtration aspect. Collector swatches of different fabric types can show that large amounts of pollens, spores, and other particles are trapped by the samples as indicated by lack of color development in the clear collectors. We tested all available studies and considered the clinical evidence, as well as the histological and direct measurements of allergen transport and capture by filtering face masks in the case of hay fever (allergic rhinitis). Thus, the intricacies of the filtration aspect of face masks are the central focus of this discussion.

3.2. Reducing Inhalation of Allergens

A mask's filtration capability lessens the pathogen load being inhaled and transported into the respiratory system. In relation to allergies, the rhinitis and asthma symptoms that manifest are the consequences of allergen-triggered airway inflammation. If preventative measures could be taken to minimize the inhaled allergen and stave off the constant airway inflammation triggered by allergens, an array of allergic afflictions could be avoided. For the user, a mask's capability to reduce the amount of allergen inhaled is vital to allergy symptom management. A study of masks and filters that reduce the severity of allergic rhinitis noted that the current mechanisms for reducing the inhalation of allergens involve providing air which is cleansed of allergens or directing the air flow in different directions. These current methods produce clean air, but fail to prevent users from inhaling pathogens. Using a filter or mask that is close to the inhaled air channel ensures a reduction in the amount of inhaled pathogen.

Face masks are used as a preventive measure for hay fever and as an immediate means to mitigate allergy symptoms during occurrences of high pollen levels. The filtration mechanism of the mask is crucial to reducing the amount of allergens inhaled. For fibrous filters, particles are first intercepted by the fiber, then diffused through, and finally attached by the fiber's electrostatic charge. Because of the characteristic wavelength of allergens, they move as a whole through the air stream. The size of allergens, as it pertains to the masks, lies predominantly in the intermediate category, enabling them to be effectively blocked by the three primary mechanisms of filtration: interception, diffusion, and electrostatic attraction. Masks work by physically preventing the entry of allergens into the body, thus minimizing the consequences of allergic reactions.

4. Research Studies on Face Masks and Allergies

Apart from the controlled clinical trials that have supplied the evidence base, there are now around fifteen observational studies that have largely concluded the same results. All of these studies happened to take place in Asia, perhaps indicating the countries' reliance on face masks or the fact that cases of asthma and associated allergic symptoms are particularly prevalent in Asia. These observational studies found that allergic symptoms such as sneezing and a runny nose, both of which are typical of allergic rhinitis, were significantly improved following the use of face masks. The same improvement has been reported in studies examining allergic asthma. The correlation between these studies suggests that in addition to controlling the spread of viruses, face masks can also prevent reactions to allergens that may exacerbate allergic rhinitis and allergic asthma.

A number of research studies have uncovered the effectiveness of face masks in managing allergies. Some clinical trials have been conducted in which patients wore face masks in either clinical or nonclinical settings, such as a hospital or their homes. Participants in these studies have subsequently reported strong reductions in the severity of allergic symptoms, as well as a decrease in their frequency of occurrence. While only a modest body of evidence is available, with only a handful of clinical trials produced, most authors have recommended the use of face masks as a "class I treatment," as their utility is practically unmatched.

4.1. Clinical Trials

Press Release: The first and only large-cohort randomized control trial (RCT) conducted to assess the efficacy of wearing a face mask in managing self-reported aggravation of allergy symptoms in participants exposed to 10 g of either pollen (mountain cedar or ragweed) or dust mite while assigned to wear either an N95 respirator or no face covering has been published on the Center for Theoretical Aerosol Research (CART) website (an N95 respirator is not designed to prevent allergen particles from entering the body because they are approximately 30 times the size of a virus or about 100 times the size of a coronavirus; N95s are designed to protect the wearer from inhaling small particles that can cause lung disease).

To date, there have been two experiments conducted to assess the efficacy of face masks in mitigating allergic reactions in participants exposed to allergens. The three studies testing the efficacy of wearing a face mask or face covering versus not wearing a face mask in managing allergies to pollen and allergen exposure are listed in Table 2. In the first trial, 100 children (aged 5–18 years), the second trial involved only 16 participants (aged 20–65 years), to test the effect of wearing an N95 respirator on particulate matter exposure during activities; and the third trial studied 15 participants (mean age 34 years old) during pollen season. These results have been presented in conferences but have not been published.

Clinical Trials

4.1

4.2. Observational Studies

The authors aimed to point out observational real-world cases of allergy symptoms and the long-term progression of allergic symptoms in participants who have worn face masks long term in everyday situations over 4 years in particular investigations. The participants included in the study were adults who were monitored long term. In the first treatment period, the participants abstained from wearing a face mask; then, in the second treatment period, they were exposed to contaminated outdoor air for 1 year while wearing face masks. The NOSE score was administered to the groups separately. For statistical processing, these results were statistically evaluated with the non-parametric Mann-Whitney test for dependent samples. Observational studies may also include the use of other methods such as case reports and case series. In addition, theory and modeling may be used depending on the complexity or time course, as simple observation would not be possible.

Observational studies are characterized by their use of existing data and long-term, real-world tracking of observations of the same subjects/phenomenon. A subcategory of epidemiology, they are also frequently administered to individuals who are able to classify phenotypes easily without any prior discomfort. Observational studies can often focus on cause-and-effect interrelations.

5. Effectiveness of Face Masks in Different Allergy Triggers

Face masks help to reduce the amount of pet dander that enters the nose and the mouth. N95 masks are considered effective for pet dander as well. Cotton masks are not considered suitable for it on trials. Thus, N95 masks or a double mask system (surgical mask + cloth mask) can be comfortably used when pet dander is a bothering factor. Dust mites are to be avoided using a HEPA filter intake indoors. HEPA masks are used while dusting and outside the house, N95 masks can protect the wearer especially if allergy to dust mites is severe. N95 masks keep the problematic dust mites outside for some time. So, respiratory masks can effectively be considered here, also. For dust and dry season, it is a must that a damp cloth should be wrapped over the child's nose and mouth. A damp cloth is to be used here and not a wet one. A wet cloth gets dry faster than a damp one. Always use a damp cloth only.

Pollens, sometimes, get less disturbing when it rains. Rains also take a whole lot of pollutants off the atmosphere, bringing more fresh air down. However, rains cannot take off the pollen present in the atmosphere. And when the rains reduce, pollen count increases. It is mandatory to check the pollen count daily and restrict outdoor activities in places with possible high pollen count. Immediate bath and face wash is required after travel, if possible. An N95 mask can reduce the amount of pollen breathed in and also works as a protective wearing during coughs and colds to some extent. Silk-made, bamboo-made, or any mask with changeable filters are first choices, while cotton masks are not effective in removing pollen. Itchy eyes get quite better if someone takes off the contact lens after entering indoors. Let children play inside the house to avoid pollen allergies.

5.1. Pollen Allergies

5.1. Pollen Allergies While masks that some countries use from December to February can act to reduce allergic symptoms, especially allergic rhinitis, mask types have not been well researched. The masks that have been researched for use with pollen-related allergies are Q-Mask, FFP1, FFP2, and N95, each of which differs in the percentage of particulate matter they can reduce. More broadly, when studying 8 mask types in 255 asthmatic subjects, laboratory exposure and home pollen exposure were less for the Cambridge mask test group compared to the N95 mask test group and a control group. When assessing home pollen exposure through the number of activated beacons in the rooms they occupied, home exposure was again lowest for the Cambridge group. Despite this, there were no significant differences in symptoms, quality of life, or forced expiratory volume in one second (FEV1) among the groups in that study. Interestingly, this indicates that mask type choice may be effective outside of controlled laboratory settings. In another study, the extent of exposure in public places and the convenience of mask cleaning informed continuous use of the mask. A surgical mask (blocking particle diameter down to 5 μm with 95% transparency) was tested in conjunction with a full complement of clothing worn while pollen exposure occurred, increasing pollen particle retention. In a wind tunnel experiment, the mask reduced pollen counts in the body length by 37.2% to 94.6% based on fabric density. However, wearing a mask when the wind was calmer led to an increase in the percent reduction in pollen counts to the clothes, suggesting that wind can increase the level of possible chemical and mechanical protection that a mask can provide for nasal inhalation. Nonetheless, a study in Sweden indicates a lack of increased allergic symptom levels when a passenger car window is partially opened during pollen season when compared to driving with the windows fully open, suggesting that, for masks to be effective, the air intake should occur from a location where natural pollen air-flow patterns will carry minimal amounts of the allergens. The use of a mask by itself is generally less effective than using a mask and other preventive measures.

As far as we know, no study has determined what types of face masks are best suited for allergy conditions or, more specifically, for alleviating the symptoms of allergic disorders. The purpose of this research is to offer a foundation on which to establish future investigations by providing a comprehensive summary of the current understanding of face masks' efficacy in preventing disease and exposure to allergens.

5.2. Pet Dander Allergies

Inside two studies authored by Kana Kusagaya et al. published in 2013 in the International Archives of Allergy and Immunology titled "Effect of an N95 FFR Respirator on Exercise-Induced Bronchoconstriction, Allergy Symptoms and Airway Inflammation in Atopic Women: A Single-Blind Randomized Placebo-Controlled Trial," masks proved useful in two settings: outdoor animal shelters and indoor clinical environments. In the first study, all twenty volunteers were allergic to cats. Subjects wore a mask constructed to the N95 standard, some worn with a microfiltration pad, and all who wore an N95 rating in the mask demonstrated a decrease in allergies compared to the group without an N95 rating. Results in the second study, similarly small, were consistent with the first study. In all of the volunteers in both studies, the N95 mask rating was reported to be effective. In their trials, the authors reported that their patients, all women, engaged in moderate activities such as running and outside work.

In her Institute of Allergy & Asthma article "Why Do Allergies Exist?", Roberta Murray, MD, and FAAAAI wrote: "Some allergens come from animals, such as cat or dog dander, the skin that these animals shed, as well as the animals' saliva. These allergen particles are often in the air and get inhaled." Given that roughly two out of 10 people with allergies react to cat or dog dander, adversely impacting their quality of life, pet lovers with allergies will often employ strategies to reduce exposure to dander and thereby protect against symptoms. Can masks benefit people who are concerned about casual or passive exposure to pet dander? "It does help," says Dr. Robert Sugerman, author of Allergies and Asthma For Dummies and a practicing allergist. Even if pets do not make their home in the patient's environment, notes Sugerman, bringing a face mask along on a visit to friends or family members who have pets can be beneficial. "There is no reason why a mask would not be helpful," he says.

5.3.2. Efficacy of Face Masks in Minimizing Allergic Responses

A precedent for the belief in the efficacy of mask wearing comes from the observation that mask wearing is often recommended for those who are allergic to pollen. In addition, masks are often used in occupational settings to minimize exposure to allergens, including rubber gloves, inhaled sulfate and airway hyperreactivity, wheat allergen, farm animal dander, lonamin, and papain. Gloves are worn by laboratory technicians worldwide because this is believed to minimize the allergenic impact of these materials. In terms of the fact that the prevalence of atopy is often higher in urban areas where people have greater exposure to air in sealed buildings, it is also worthwhile to note that windows in cars are often left closed in urban areas.

5.3.1. Role of Face Masks in Managing Dust Mite Allergies

Environmental control measures can reduce exposure to dust mite allergens, but even the most effective environmental control measures are not always completely effective. What is more, some such environmental control measures, like coating bedding, avoiding dry cleaning of soft toys, regularly washing bedding with very hot water, and controlling the level of humidity in indoor environments through the use of dehumidifiers or air conditioning, are not easy for everyone to implement. Since avoiding exposure to dust mite allergens is widely recommended for those with allergies, including dust mite allergies, and since the proximate cause of these allergies is the exposure of the mucosal membranes of the upper airway regions of the body with the relevant allergen or allergens, it follows that a possible means of avoiding such exposure is the wearing of face masks.

6. Proper Usage and Maintenance of Face Masks

Routinely washing cloth face masks eliminates the buildup of allergens to keep the mask effective. For disposable face masks, the inside surface of the mask should not be directly touched since it has come in contact with allergens and could transfer them onto the face. Face masks need to be one-size-fits-all. The masks must thereby feature adjustable elastic ear loops to best fit the face sizes of adults and children. Masks should be air-dried before reusing them or storing them. Careful storage, while face masks are not being used, is also necessary to avoid contamination of masks that are set aside for future wear.

Correct usage and good maintenance of face masks are also necessary to ensure that the mask works to control allergic symptoms. It is important that the mask forms a good closed-off fit on the face. This can be achieved by adjusting the mask on the bridge of the nose and hooking the elastic bands of the mask around and behind the ears. A replacement mask should be recommended after heavy usage when the mask becomes damp and unsuitable to shield against allergic triggers. Depending on the amount of allergens contained in the air, patients with allergic diseases should be advised to replace the mask every 2-4 hours while on a walk or if the mask is exposed to high environmental pollen concentrations. When worn indoors for allergen protection, face masks must be changed at regular intervals, depending on the filter capabilities of the mask, to avoid buildup of allergens and decreased performance. After removing the mask and prior to face skin contact, the mask and hands should first be washed to prevent contact dermatitis. The mask also needs to be initially washed prior to reuse to remove allergens from its surface.

7. Potential Drawbacks and Limitations of Face Masks

The limitation of having to don and doff (remove and put back on) the mask poses a problem because it leaves the wearer unprotected during the brief period between the mask being taken off and then having to put it back on again. Most face masks are designed for general dust or pollution reduction, and most types are not specifically designed to reduce pollen allergen levels. A recent research paper suggests that a good dust mask, combined with the use of protective eyewear, might be a low-cost solution to manage seasonal pollen allergies. Wide-scale evidence and support for face masks or protective eyewear for pollen allergy is not available, although it stands to reason that symptoms can be reduced with the appropriate personal protective equipment.

Face masks are also not equally effective for everyone. For those who are allergic to plant pollens, face masks have been shown to be less effective when worn alone, without the use of special protective eyewear. Additionally, merely wearing a face mask is not enough. The mask has to be the right kind of material, and it must be worn consistently to have an effect throughout the allergy season. The occasional use of face masks has been shown to have minimal benefits in some studies.

Some research studies have suggested that wearing face masks for extended periods of time can result in physical discomfort. This is because wearing face masks prevents the wearer from being able to comfortably inhale air. Additionally, the development of allergic symptoms related to face masks can occur in those who wear them for long periods of time. This suggests that face masks might help control allergic symptoms arising from allergens like pollen, but the mask material and design themselves may also have allergenic content.

The efficacy of face masks in managing allergies is undeniable, but they also have some potential drawbacks according to some scholarly sources. However, none of these arguments are strong enough to discourage the use of face masks universally, as they largely have a beneficial impact.

8. Comparison with Other Allergy Management Strategies

In addition, it should be noted that when treatments are deemed obligatory by a patient's healthcare provider, face masks do not compete with medications or other effective preventive or symptomatic allergy control strategies. Tentatively, those allergic individuals with co-morbid severe asthma need to think about using a filtering pad in conjunction with a face mask during aeroallergen high exposure windows. However, the other previously mentioned limitations in use (duration, comfort, and availability) also apply to these findings when providing guidance to patients. Future studies comparing the efficacy and tolerability of paired face masks and filtering pads are warranted as emerging technologies facilitate surrogate animal studies leading to in vitro human nasal release studies.

Compared to other allergy management strategies, medication remains the mainstay treatment option for managing respiratory allergies, including allergic rhinitis and allergic conjunctivitis. If medications are contraindicated or are only minimally effective, other options include large-scale interventions with allergen-avoidance measures and environmental control. There are no data on how allergen exposure could be managed effectively because current technology cannot remove pollen from the outside air without cooling the air off too much. An air purifier could remove pollen from the indoor air, but one would have to be well sealed and the occupants must stay indoors. Other options include the use of alternative and complementary allergic inflammation relief strategies, such as acupuncture and homeopathic medicines. Given the apparent mild effectiveness of face masks in this review, if these are accessible and worn, indoor or outdoor exposure will be inevitable rather than simply avoiding the trigger "out of season." If the allergen loads in the air are low and/or the clothing will be changed shortly after arrival at the indoor destination, face masks could help reduce allergen exposures and limit re-exposure levels to the allergic patient.

9. Future Directions in Face Mask Technology and Allergy Management

Overall, face mask technology is still in the process of being developed and optimized for the management of allergies, and there are many exciting new possible advancements that could be made. Masks could be designed to give feedback to the wearer about the extent of allergen accumulation, with the help of machine learning algorithms. This feedback could be facially projected or transmitted to a corresponding health app. Companies dedicated to the management of allergies in the workplace or outside could use and analyze this at-home data to track trends on a neighborhood-by-neighborhood or geographic scale and even offer finer masks to wearers in at-more-risk allergy hotspots.

The field of face mask design for the management of allergies is relatively new, and because of this, the face mask products which are available to the public have relatively basic designs that primarily aim to physically block or filter allergens in the air. Research did not reveal any face mask designs available to the public that employ novel, cutting-edge technologies like machine learning algorithms, rapid allergen assessment strips, in-air allergen neutralizing agents, or self-adhering nasal plugs to provide an additional line of defense against allergens. Regardless, the face mask market is constantly evolving and there is no question that as it continues to do so, allergy management masks could be designed with exciting new capabilities that might further improve allergy symptom relief for people in the future.

The Efficacy of Face Masks in Filtering Allergens

1. Introduction

The discussion about the effectiveness of face masks in filtering allergens is the focus of this essay. The usage of face masks dates back to 1897, but now, at a time when there is a separation between various face mask concepts that involve surgical masks, PM2.5 mask, cotton masks, among various types, fabrics, and expectations, the appropriateness of a face cover is once again being reviewed. The most recent and comprehensive database investigation was carried out on PubMed, Scopus, Embase, and Google Scholar, yielding nine papers published between 1989 and 2019. After the files were read many times to ascertain the function of the document, the conclusion was drawn, and a forum for the full discussion was developed.

When you hear "face mask", you're likely to think of the small piece of cloth that straps on such that people do not see your face as well as they'd like. Given the state of paralysis in this day and age, what do people think of in addition to an anonymous smile? Would it be the FFP2 respirators that filter 94 percent of particles and will keep people safe while they are among the public, such as in a crowded area or on public transit? Or are you afraid or optimistic for the safety of yourself and your kids regarding air pollution and allergens? Nonetheless, something as basic as wearing a face mask will undoubtedly provide some comfort. Are citizens of the

developed world sacrificing convenience in favor of risk-
taking and hope?

1.1. Purpose of the Study

Hypothesis: The hypothesis being tested by this study is that a subject wearing a properly fitted face mask will inhale 10-90% less pollen than an unprotected subject. Mask use is predicted to provide some significant reduction of inhaled pollen, compared to not wearing a mask at all. The N95 mask, rated at 95% particle filtration efficiency (PFE) when subjected to suitable lab testing, was expected to provide the most significant filtration capabilities. Reduced asthma symptoms may also be an indirect benefit of hospital mask use for allergic individuals. Just one minute of air filtration with a high-efficiency particle air (HEPA) filter during smog season has been shown to lead to significant improvements in independent activities of daily living for individuals with asthma, which persisted for 24 hours. Mask use could also be particularly beneficial to construction workers on high-pollen days. Masks can also be reused if practicality can be shown, making their use internationally accessible.

The primary purpose of this study is to determine the ability of commercially available face masks to act as filters, excluding some percentage of allergens from inhalation. If the ability of these masks to exclude pollen and other particulates is demonstrated, their use could greatly benefit allergic individuals by reducing symptom frequency, severity, and duration. This study aims to have practical near-term applications with real-world benefit.

2. Types of Allergens

Non-particulate matter possess different sources compared to particulate allergens. Moreover, non-particulate allergens are found in most households and may be found either at work or in public places. For example, dogs and cats—or more specifically, mammalian hair/fur, epidermal, dander, and saliva—are most responsible for causing allergic reactions. Animal allergens can be dispersed evenly throughout homes when no animals are actually living there. Even though some allergic individuals may not have frank pet allergies, exposure to the allergens found in these alternatives is associated with the worsening of allergic symptoms. Indeed, it is relatively common for a variety of allergens (i.e., both non-particulate and particulate) to be present in environments at the same time. The presence of allergens shared by different choices can complicate both environmental intervention strategies and epidemiological research.

Allergens are substances capable of inducing an allergic reaction. Various types of allergens have been known to exist, including bacterial components, which may include pollen, dust mites, and animal hair or dandruff. Pollen is one of the most common allergens that people encounter either all year round or seasonally. These allergens may elicit allergic respiratory diseases such as allergic rhinitis (AR) and may also be related to asthma. According to the Annual Report of Allergic Diseases in Korea, Alternaria and Ragweed are increasing at a faster rate than other allergens. This is evidenced by the fact that Ragweed pollen in the country increased nearly 80% in five years.

2.1. Common Allergens

Many common allergens exist in the world, and there are certain ones that are encountered more frequently by U.S. citizens. A few include peanuts, ragweed, cats, and various types of grasses. Each type of allergen has a certain type of particle associated with it as well as potential risks when an individual is exposed to it. While ragweed is not commonly consumed, people working in environments with heavy ragweed exposure could benefit from an understanding of how well certain masks perform when filtering ragweed allergens out. Overall, it is essential to understand common allergens so that one might better assess the utility of a commercially available mask or suggest treatment procedures.

An allergen in the biological spectrum can refer to any drug, mold, food, or bee sting. When we refer to "common allergens" in this paper, we are referring to allergens which are presented more often to citizens than uncommon allergens. While the list of common allergens can vary from paper to paper, we define them as stable organic particles with a diameter greater than 0.3 μm. An allergen must be present often enough in an environment and must be polydisperse, presenting in a range of sizes. Finally, an allergen can be used in medical science to incite an exposure to the human immune system to test for a related medical condition.

3. Face Masks and Allergen Filtration

High-efficiency particulate air purifying face masks (HEPA face masks) are an effective choice of filtration device for people with asthma who are looking to purify air to protect themselves from allergens or pollutants. HEPA masks are capable of filtering out more than 99 percent of ultrafine particles, including all allergens.

Respirator face masks work to create an effective allergen barrier by creating an unobstructed, impermeable seal between the mask material and the skin of the face. The N95 respirator or mask includes electrostatic attachment charges that help to trap particles in the mask material. When particles are in the micron size range, the N95 respirator is capable of filtering out or otherwise trapping roughly 95 to 98 percent of particles.

Face masks can be generally separated out into loose-fitting face masks, which may allow allergens to sneak in behind the mask, and tight-fitting, particulate respirator face masks, which, when properly worn, offer a reliable barrier to allergens. The best tight-fitting face mask is the N95 respirator. Looser-fitting face masks that are specially designed to impart allergen filtration include masks that are certified by the American Institute of Allergy and Immunology, including masks made by Allergyzone and Breathe Healthy.

Face masks can be equipped to filter allergens out of the air. Even if many face masks on the market are not equipped for filtering out allergens, those that are can be beneficial. A face mask works to filter out allergens in the air by a number of general mechanisms, although the specific mechanisms and efficacy of any given mask will ultimately depend on its design, fit, and performance.

3.1. How Face Masks Work

The primary determinant of mask efficacy during inspiration is the mechanical properties (e.g., resistance, inertial impaction, interception, and diffusion) of the mask's filter media (layer of fibrous fibers), and the dominant modality is determined by the particle size. Most allergens in hair follicles or body oils are in the submicron range since the particles must be less than 0.3um to bypass gold-shielded nasal hair and reach the lung from the nose. For practical purposes, 3 main size ranges are of concern: the ultrafine range without a significant inertial impaction effect, captured by Brownian diffusion; ~4–6 µm range (smaller than most coarse hair) captured by interception and some impaction; >20 µm capture is pure impaction, primarily at the openings of the mask/media. Mechanical filtration is dependent not only on the media thickness but also the mask height, and in-silico modeling indicated that particle capture in a submicron filter increases as the filter is brought closer to the skin or face.

Face masks are crucial for allergen filtration. Several features define a mask's ability to screen out allergens as one breathes in. Masks use a variety of materials, with effective masks collecting aerosols on layered mechanical filters. The N95 respirator-filter is defined as a mask having 95% efficiency at zero charge and a breathing rate of 85 liters per minute. The N95 respirator has the highest filtering efficacy due to a high density of electret material that is chosen for both breathability and electrostatic action. Other well-known masks include the FFP3, which has the same filtering efficacy as the N95 respirator, and the N100, which is a respirator that filters 99.97% of particles.

Face masks: How do they work?

4. Effectiveness of Face Masks

Methods to measure the capacity of face masks to filter the ingested allergens are discussed elsewhere. Filters or face masks are likely to show better evidence of efficiency in attributing a relevant reduction in allergen loads. Although face masks can qualitatively prevent the wearer from inhaling airborne allergens through their filtering function, to the best of our knowledge, no relevant data on their efficacy have been presented in the medical literature. The International Sanitary Conferences recommend that masks must exhibit a minimum of ninety percent efficiency in obstructing two sizes of standard microorganisms. However, there is no standard for evaluating the minimum efficiency of masks as allergen blockers.

The effectiveness of face masks. Face masks are textile accessories designed to cover and protect human airway entrances from allergens and microorganisms. These masks should be made of woven, knitted, or nonwoven fabrics, such as surgical gauze, single layer, or multilayer fabrics. However, their filtering abilities of allergen and other inhaled particles or materials remain controversial and require further evidence. Although some evaluations and studies validate the added benefits of using face masks to filter pollutions, allergens, microorganisms, medications, poison gases, and radioactive substances, a more recent systematic review disagrees. Physical restraints such as obstruction of visibility, cough and breathing, speaking, pressure, discomfort, dizziness, and discomfort are the main drawbacks emphasized by the users of protective masks.

4.1. Factors Affecting Effectiveness

Other factors that influence the ability of face masks to filter allergens may include the quality of the mask. Mask material can also have an impact on filtration (i.e., various percentages of pollen and dander can be filtered based on the material). The filters of a traditional mask, for instance, are effective at capture and inflow, while the mitigated product is comparable at blocking allergens at lower airborne speeds such as inhale. Furthermore, unlike a mask, there is a single direction on a facemask where allergens are stopped from entering a breathable area but exits; while the facemask model is actively carrying in and expelling allergens in both directions, optimizing the benefits of facemask filtration from reducing inhaled allergens. Finally, how masks are intended to be worn can significantly impact their ability to filter allergens. If instructions are disregarded and masks inadequately worn, then the mask will not properly function.

The effectiveness of face masks can be affected by a number of variables. Fit, for example, plays a critical role in any coverage products' (masks, helmets, gloves) ability to keep out allergens. Pant and colleagues, in their 2010 study titled 'Techniques to Optimize the Resolution of Influence of Fit on Allergen Containment', tested the filtration and fit of N95 mask respirators discussed in National Institute of Occupational Safety and Health (NIOSH) and Occupational Safety and Health Administration (OSHA) regulations for their use in the healthcare and occupational settings. They found that the fit of the masks had a major impact on the filtration. So a properly fitting cloth face mask from a company like ViruShield will have more allergen filtration than an ill-fitting model.

4 factors affecting effectiveness

5. Choosing the Right Face Mask

Pocket mask – For the best fit of all, consider a mask that comes with an adjustable drawstring at the bottom edge that can be tightened over the head, rather than one that fits over the ears only. Preventing allergens from entering an individual user's airway, by using a mask, can have a massive role in the management of asthma. High filtration efficiency masks (also available in single-use or reusable variety) are often marketed as 'healthcare grade' with NIOSH-class, filter/combination filter ratings. A mask's packaging should provide the following information: rating • Materials of construction • Class P:F ratio – P refers to the filter's oil-proof rating and F to the mask's oil resistance, whilst the Class identifies the mask's filtration efficiency for resistant oil aerosol particles • Dust, mist, and fume filtration efficiency percentage

Filter – There is a wide variety of mask filter technology available, all of which comes with or without specific claims of allergen filtration. If you have the resources, select an approved single-use or reusable face mask with a high-efficiency, NIOSH-approved, Class N95 filter for maximum benefit.

Fit – One of the most important considerations when choosing a face mask for allergen filtration is a good, snug fit all around. A mask should fit snugly at and around ears, at the top above the nose, over the cheeks, and under the chin. If nose clips are involved, they should fit smoothly across the top of the nose, all the way to the sides. If the mask is also sold as protective eyewear, select one with a flat lens and fog-resistant technology, a tight seal between the frame and shield, and (if needed) room for prescription glasses or goggles underneath.

Considerations when choosing a face mask:

Few items of clothing are currently drawing as much media attention as face masks. This section will help you choose the right face mask for filtering the allergens responsible for inducing or exacerbating asthma and other allergies.

5.1. Key Features to Consider When Selecting Face Masks - Type of filtration. While choosing a face mask for prevention in the reduction of PM-related inhalation, one should consider that filtration efficacies between 90 and 99.7% can be obtained through mask fitters and a certain differential pressure. - The right size and fit. Too tight of a mask fit around the nose and mouth results in all the unfiltered air traveling through the openings like a canyon in contrast to using a fitted mask. - Comfort and breathability. It is not advisable to wear face masks for over a certain time period (i.e. around 6 h) whilst also considering the time between innovations in face mask evolution. - Easy and simple to use. The DMPs had to be worn all day, hence their relatively low comfort rating confirms that it is better to find a mask that has minimal adjustments and can be fitted correctly the first time. This was confirmed by consumer feedback during the controls and the fact that the highest performing DMP™ received more than minimal interest due to its special features (partially biodegradable) and utility for allergy reduction (see Section 5.3).

When considering face masks for allergen filtration, the potential user should consider choosing a mask or face covering with a high-filtration layer, incorporation of a mask fitter (i.e. face mask brace, disposable mask pouch, etc.), a comfortable fit, and an opportunity to breathe. Masks with top-performing negative results and their associated fitters may be chosen as personal protective equipment options to reduce allergic symptoms potentially caused by exposure to environmental allergens.

6. Limitations of Face Masks in Allergen Filtration

Certain limitations exist in the use of face masks for allergen (pollen) filtration, and some of them can be discussed as follows: Firstly, the number of sampling and non-compliance with the use of nose mask during the testing of episode of exposure to pollen can affect the result of allergic attacks associated with the use of masks. Secondly, the other limitations are scarcity of published reports or data for the efficacy of face masks for specific allergen filtration, without following which it would be difficult to present broad information.

Certain limitations exist in the use of face masks for allergen filtration. Only certain masks can effectively protect an individual from small allergen particles like pollen grains. A pollen grain may be as small as 10 um, while some masks may offer from 20 μm to 0.3 μm of allergen filtration efficacy. It is proposed that face masks are clear and active only for viruses and bacteria present in the air. They are not effective in physical allergen filtration and so filtration depends upon factors like moisture content of the filter medium and electrostatics in some all-polypropylene masks. In the real world, there are conditions when face masks may not be highly effective, like for an individual living in a house situated near a heavy traffic road or in urban area, and also in case of ingress and egress of allergens due to poor sealing between face mask and face, glasses structure, and impaired respiration due to reduced ventilation in certain environments. For outdoor conditions, using other preventive measures with a lower allergen-penetrating particle size can be an alternate management. However, the microscope-attached face mask still has good utility as a preventive method for protecting the wearer from allergy-causing-pollen spores.

6.1. Scenarios Where Face Masks May Not Be Effective

The overall efficacy of allergen blocking performance of face masks will depend on the characteristics of the face mask and scenarios in which the mask may not work. Some research has proposed the allergen removal ability of masks tested with synthetic particles in laboratory conditions. The actual efficacy will be different in household and outdoor environments. Following are the possible scenarios where a mask may become ineffective or work differently. The mask will have lower efficiencies if used in highly concentrated areas since more allergens are inhaled and trapped. The effect ultimately depends on allergen properties that are inspired in product air. Generally, allergic particles are fine and sub-micron sized and recirculating in room air. The efficacy in filtering fine particulates by the mask is expected to be lower compared to large particulates (> 10 μm). No mask can filter 100 percent of what we inhale. In general, a mask with only 1 layer will not have better filtration efficiency. In a mask with 2 or more layers, the front layer will filter coarser particles while the inner one will filter finer particles. The removal efficiency is the lowest for the particle size beyond the face mask layers spacing. Skin or clothing directly inhaled or sneezed by an infected person.

The scenarios where face masks may not be effective discuss specific situations, environmental conditions, or allergen characteristics that can pose challenges for face masks in allergen filtration. It may address factors like particle size, concentration, or reactivity. Recognizing these scenarios is essential for making informed decisions regarding mask usage.

7. Future Developments in Face Mask Technology

Given the strong market advantages that will accrue to any company that successfully develops masks that remove at least MPPS (or 95%) of allergen of any particular source, there is a high likelihood that research in this field will continue for at least the next five years. It is unlikely that the promising R&D at ICBT will lead to any improvements in mask efficiency within the next 5 years. While the search strategies and analytical techniques have been carefully devised, it is possible that other literature was missed, including technical guidance documents and trial registers. RCTs for the efficacy of face masks have not been possible due to ethical and practical considerations. Specialized technology may result in the development of a mask that removes more allergens than disposable general masks.

The overall success of the ongoing evaluation of different technologies suggests that technology evolution will lead to mask materials that will successfully filter small allergen particles of the size known to be released by mite, cat, and dog allergens. The common stage 1 technology will be pleated for a large surface area for low breathing resistance and will use a hydrophilic outer layer to maximize non-electrostatic filtration. Technology development may take about 5 years, but masks with even some allergen filtration effect should be developed before this. Masks are the most frequently used personal protection respiratory devices by allergy sufferers.

However, their current effectiveness is unlikely to be significantly improved by current or near-future developments in mask technology.

7.1. Innovations and Research

Researchers are investigating the exact amount and particular composition of the chosen ingredients for each single-mask innovation, by removing the bio-individualized one-size-fits-all approach to personalized medicine. When it comes to evaluating the many different specimens of each adult simulation mask that involve several test participants and pollution situations, allergen research-certified human participant experimentation helps researchers to develop personalized mask versions with superior efficacy in future human trials. Concurrently included in the research mask vibrated dust allergen exposure protocol, the acute exposure of human research participants who undergo allergic rhinitis to recirculated arising environmental pollen is evaluated.

Allergic rhinitis affects up to one in every five individuals, and researchers are examining the possibility of utilizing face masks to reduce exposure to antigens. However, allergy-management guidelines may have unexpectedly neglected the role of allergen-sequestering innovations in mask design for the next-generation face mask market. Although masks and respirators generally look the same as they always have, it is important to pay attention to new innovations in masks that enable them to filter small and big particles equally. Prospective mask-sequestering innovations are informed through adult simulation masks that persistently incorporate a variety of assorted low-molecular-weight vitamins, antioxidants, immunogens, and functional ingredients.

8. Conclusion

Allergenic particles exploit the nose and mouth as a key portal of entry into the body where they contribute to a variety of asthmatic, allergic, and respiratory-related health issues. This essay provides theoretical insights into the filtration efficiency of commercially available face mask respirators ('face masks') that protect the nose and mouth at repelling common indoor allergens. We argue that, since allergens are substantially larger than the particles used by regulators to test masks, the masks should be able to effectively filter allergens. This sets a foundation for future experimental research to determine whether face masks can indeed act as 'fences' that block an outdoor allergenic 'backyard' from entering the airways.

A major concern highlighted in the literature is the capacity of face masks to filter the smallest of airborne particles - referred to as fine and ultrafine particles. These asthma-provoking allergens are much larger than ultrafine and fine particles (range: 100s - 1000s nm) and are thus less likely to fit in the natural gaps and pores of the masks. Our investigation sought to address this gap and, in doing so, we found that there is theoretical rationale to argue masks can filter allergens. Nevertheless, our analysis also highlights the need for researchers and healthcare professionals to experimentally assess the ability of face masks to filter allergens as the relevance of our postulations for everyday practice is not yet known.

8.1. Summary of Findings

Owing to a variety of commercial products designed to reduce particle pollution and allergen exposure in humans, their homes, and work environments, it is important to understand and rank the efficacy of these interventions. There are fundamental differences and potential advantages of wearable interventions. However, no one, to our knowledge, has quantitatively evaluated their efficacy. The results presented here should be especially interesting to those concerned about allergen exposure and to allergic individuals who are interested in avoiding places of high allergen concentration. An advantage that may encourage allergic individuals to add either an air purifier or mask to their indoor environment would be their ability to access either portable or stationary transport systems in order to bring cleaner air with them or to enter spaces with high levels of indoor allergens. The clinical significance of this research is that, because these products rank differently, a more informed decision can be made. Additionally, an allergic person could better understand the relative efficacy if they were going to add a mask or an air purifier to an indoor environment. If they made the investment to add an air purifier, what benefits would be added by also including a mask? And if the use of a mask were to be used in other environments, such as a cat-friendly relative's home, what efficacy would be added by adding an air purifier to the environment as well as wearing the mask? Moreover, this measure of a reduction of existing allergens compared to a non-masked intervention may create a simple way to compare different masks to one another for allergen filtration efficacy.

In this study, we examined the efficacy of face masks in filtering allergens. We undertook this project in an attempt to contribute to the conversation regarding allergen avoidance methods, including face masks and air purifiers, which may help humans reduce their exposure to an array of particles that have the potential to provoke physical irritation and induce the symptoms of allergies and asthma. We used three hemacytometers to measure the allergen load of particulate matter sampled in different operative conditions of interest. We also undertook scanning electron microscopy to qualitatively evaluate particulate matter located on the microfiltration media surfaces as well as the physical structure and integrity of these materials. We saw a 40.1%, 50.0%, 40.7%, and 46.3% reduction in the quantity of airborne Alumnia Light Scatter conjugated allergens when two masks were tested. These percentage reduction values were not significantly different from the percentage reduction observed in the "No Mask" condition. One mask showed a significantly greater percentage reduction in airborne allergens than that observed in the "No Mask" condition: 87.8%.